DISCOVERING
CAREERS FOR YOUR FUTURE

health

Ferguson Publishing Company
Chicago, Illinois

Carol Yehling
Editor

Beth Adler, Herman Adler Design Group
Cover design

Carol Yehling
Interior design

Laurie Sabol
Proofreader

Library of Congress Cataloging-in-Publication Data

Discovering careers for your future. Health.
          p. cm.
    Includes index.
    Summary: Describes the education, training, earnings, and outlook associated with twenty careers in the field of health, including chiropractor, dentist, fitness expert, hospice worker, medical secretary, nurse, physical therapist, and physician.
    ISBN 0-89434-322-X
    1. Medicine—Vocational guidance—Juvenile literature. [1. Medicine—Vocational guidance. 2. Vocational guidance.] I. Title: Health

R690.D55 2000
610.69—dc21

                                                                                    00-020939

Published and distributed by
Ferguson Publishing Company
200 West Jackson Boulevard, 7th Floor
Chicago, Illinois 60606
800-306-9941
www.fergpubco.com

Table of Contents

Photo Credits

Advanced Practice Nurses, p. 7, *Carle Foundation Hospital, Urbana, IL*

Biomedical Engineers, p. 11, *Wright State University*

Chiropractors, p. 15, *Life Chiropractic College*

Dental Hygienists, p. 19, *American Dental Association*

Home Health Care Aides, p. 39, *Carle Foundation Hospital, Urbana, IL*

Medical Secretaries, p. 51, *Covenant Medical Center, Champaign, IL*

Medical Technologists, p. 55, *Carle Foundation Hospital, Urbana, IL*

Nurse Assistants, p. 59, *Carle Foundation Hospital,* Urbana, IL

Nurses, p. 63, *Mathew Hohmann*

Nutritionists, p. 67, *Carle Foundation Hospital,* Urbana, IL

Orthotists and Prosthetists, p. 71, *Orthotics and Prosthetics National Office*

Physical Therapists, p. 75, *Covenant Medical Center, Champaign, IL*

Physicians, p. 79, *Carle Foundation Hospital,* Urbana, IL

Introduction

You may not have decided yet what you want to be in the future. And you don't have to decide right away. You do know that right now you are interested in medicine and health care. Do any of the statements below describe you? If so, you may want to begin thinking about what a career in health care might mean for you.

___ Science is my favorite subject in school.

___ I like to do science experiments.

___ I like health class.

___ I am interested in nutrition.

___ I like to take care of people.

___ I like to help people with disabilities.

___ I am interested in the human body and how it works.

___ I collect specimens to view under my microscope.

___ I am curious about how things work.

___ I am good at observing small details.

___ I would like to find a cure for cancer or AIDS.

___ I like to babysit my younger brothers and sisters.

___ I am interested in learning first aid and CPR.

___ Physical fitness and proper diet are important to me.

Health: Discovering Careers for Your Future is a book about careers in health care and medicine, from advanced practice nurses to physicians. The health care field is growing rapidly. Health care workers are employed in hospitals, clinics, medical offices, hospices, and nursing homes. They also work in schools, universities, research labs, pharmaceutical companies, cosmetic companies, food processing plants, and in all types of industry making sure other workers stay safe and healthy.

This book describes many possibilities for future careers in medicine and health care. Read through it and see how different careers are connected. For example, if you are interested in nursing, you will want to read the chapters on Advanced Practice Nurses, Nurses, Nurse Assistants, Home Health Care Aides, and Hospice Workers. If you are interested in technical careers, you will want to read the chapters on Biomedical Engineers, Emergency Medical Technicians, Medical Record Technicians, and Medical Technologists. Go ahead and explore!

What do they do?

The first section of each chapter begins with a heading such as "What Chiropractors Do" or "What Fitness Experts Do." It tells what it's like to work at this job. It describes typical responsibilities and assignments. You will find out about working conditions. Which health care professionals work in laboratories? Which ones work with patients? What tools and equipment do they use? This section answers all these questions.

How do I get there?

The section called "Education and Training" tells you what schooling you need for employment in each job—a high school diploma, training at a junior college, a college degree, or more. It also talks about on-the-job training that you could expect to receive after you're hired and whether or not you must complete an apprenticeship program.

How much do they earn?

The "Earnings" section gives the average salary figures for the job described in the chapter. These figures provide you with a general idea of how much money people with this job can make. Keep in mind that many people really earn more or less than the amounts given here because actual salaries depend on many different things, such as the size of the company, the location of the company, and the amount of education, training, and experience you have. Generally, but not always, bigger companies located in major cities pay more than smaller ones in smaller cities and towns, and people with more education, training and experience earn more. Also remember that these figures are current averages. They will probably be different by the time you are ready to enter the workforce.

What will the future be like for health careers?

The "Outlook" section discusses the employment outlook for the career: whether the total number of people employed in this career will increase or decrease in the coming years and whether jobs in this field will be easy or hard to find. These predictions are based on economic conditions, the size and makeup of the population, foreign competition, and new technology. Keep in mind that these predictions are general statements. No one knows for sure what the future will be like. Also remember that the employment outlook is a general statement about an industry and does not necessarily apply to everyone. A determined and talented person may be able to find a job in an industry or career with the worst kind of outlook. And a person without ambition and the proper training will find it difficult to find a job in even a booming industry or career field.

Where can I find more information?

Each chapter includes a sidebar called "For More Information." It lists organizations that you can contact to find out more about the field and careers in the field. You will find names, addresses, phone numbers, and Web sites.

Extras

Every chapter has a few extras. There are photos that show scientists in action. There are sidebars and notes on ways to explore the field, related jobs, fun facts, profiles of people in the field, or lists of Web sites and books that might be helpful. At the end of the book you will find a glossary, which gives brief definitions of words that relate to education, career training, or employment that you may be unfamiliar with. There is an index of all the job titles mentioned in the book, followed by a list of health Web sites.

It's not too soon to think about your future. We hope you discover several possible career choices. Happy hunting!

Advanced Practice Nurses

What Advanced Practice Nurses Do

Advanced Practice Nurses (A.P.N.s) are registered nurses (R.N.s) who have advanced training. There are four types of A.P.N.s: nurse practitioners, certified nurse-midwives, nurse anesthetists, and clinical nurse specialists.

Nurse practitioners specialize in pediatric, adult, or family care. Nurse practitioners have many duties. They conduct physicals, diagnose and treat common illnesses, and order tests and X rays. In some states they can even prescribe prescription drugs. They regularly report a patient's treatment plan to a physician. They often send patients to physicians for further care or treatment.

Certified nurse-midwives provide care to expectant mothers and to women with gynecological problems. They work under the supervision of obstetricians. C.N.M.s teach pregnant women about

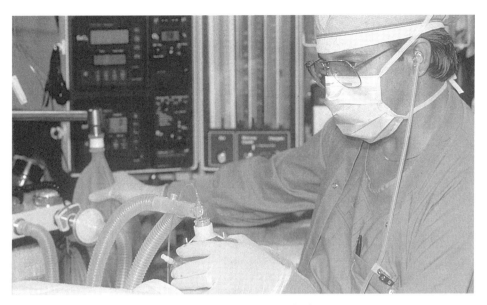

A nurse anesthetist gives anesthesia to a patient before surgery.

proper diet and predelivery health practices. They monitor the general health of expectant mothers to make sure that healthy babies will be delivered. C.N.M.s, with the help of physicians, deliver babies. Then they monitor and instruct mothers and babies after the birth.

Nurse anesthetists give patients medication for pain (anesthetics) or to help patients relax and sleep (sedatives). Some may work in dentists' offices. Nurse anesthetists may give anesthetics in a shot, or they may use gas equipment and have the patient breathe in the anesthetic through a mask. During the operation, nurse anesthetists keep track of how deeply the patient is sleeping. If the

EXPLORING

• Take a first aid class.

• Offer to care for a sick grandparent or elderly neighbor.

• Offer to babysit your younger sisters and brothers or other children in your neighborhood.

patient starts to wake up during the operation, nurse anesthetists may give more anesthetic. They closely watch a patient's breathing and heartbeat during the whole operation. In emergencies, during surgery, or during the delivery of babies, they may have to make important decisions very quickly.

ALPHABET SOUP

ACNM	American College of Nurse-Midwives
APN	Advanced Practice Nurse
CNM	Certified Nurse-Midwife
CNS	Certified Nurse Specialist
CPM	Certified Professional Midwife
CRNA	Certified Registered Nurse Anesthetist
FNP	Family Nurse Practitioner
HMO	Health Maintenance Organization
LPN	Licensed Practical Nurse
NARM	North American Registry of Midwives
PA	Physician Assistant
PND	Pediatric Nurse Practitioner
RN	Registered Nurse

Clinical nurse specialists handle many physical and mental health problems. They use patients' medical records, laboratory test results, and examinations to diagnose and treat illnesses. In addition to working directly with patients, C.N.S.s act as consultants, do research, and sometimes teach.

Education and Training

If you are interested in becoming an advanced practice nurse you must first become an R.N. To become an R.N., you must complete high school. Then you must have one of three types of training: an associate's degree, a diploma program, or a bachelor's degree. After your R.N. program, you must pass a state licensing exam.

After you become an R.N., there are a wide variety of requirements for the different types of advanced practice nurses. A master's degree is usually required, along with specific certification depending on the specialty.

Earnings

Salaries (including overtime and on-call pay) vary greatly for A.P.N.s. Salaries for nurse practitioners average about $50,000 a year. C.N.M.s average about $70,000 a year. Nurse anesthetists average $86,000 a year. C.N.S.s average $47,000 a year. A.P.N.s enjoy other benefits such as paid vacations, holidays, and sick days, health insurance, and retirement plans.

FOR MORE INFO

For more information on training programs and financial assistance, write to:
American Nurses' Association
600 Maryland Avenue, SW, Suite 100W
Washington, DC 20024-2571
Tel: 800-274-4ANA
Web: http://www.nursingworld.org

National Alliance of Nurse Practitioners
325 Pennsylvania Avenue, SE
Washington, DC 20003-1100
Tel: 202-675-6350

Where Do A.P.N.s Work?

• Community health centers
• Public health departments
• Hospitals and hospital clinics
• School and college student health clinics
• Business and industry employee health departments
• Physicians' offices
• Health maintenance organizations
• Nursing homes and hospices
• Home health agencies
• Armed forces and veteran's administration facilities
• Schools of nursing

Outlook

In the next decade, opportunities for well-trained advanced practice nurses will be very good. They have the training to perform some of the duties that doctors usually do. This gives doctors more time to treat difficult cases. Doctors will rely more and more on A.P.N.s in the future.

Biomedical Engineers

What Biomedical Engineers Do

Biomedical engineers are scientists who study how living things work. Some biomedical engineers do research in laboratories. They work with other scientists and medical doctors to learn more about all the different systems that keep people and animals alive. For example, they may study how the brain uses electrical energy or what chemicals help a plant cell make food. They use complex machines and instruments to take measurements and test new ideas. Computers help biomedical engineers figure out how living things will react to new circumstances.

Other biomedical engineers design machines, such as heart pacemakers, that will help people with health problems. These biomedical design engineers use all they know about the human body to make artificial body parts that will work as well as the real ones. For example, artificial limbs that respond to the electri-

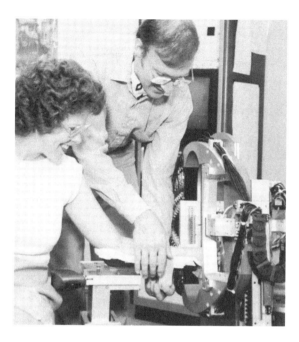

cal impulses of nerves can have fingers and toes that move exactly as they would in the natural limb.

Biomedical engineers also design machines and instruments that doctors can use to treat patients. For example, biomedical engineers work on machines that bounce sound waves to give doctors a picture of what's inside a person's body. These machines are called ultrasonic imagery devices.

Some biomedical engineers are university teachers. They lecture in classrooms and show students how to use equipment and perform experiments in the laboratory. They also teach students how to perform

EXPLORING

• Visit school and community libraries to find books written about careers in medical technology.

• Join a hobby club devoted to chemistry, biology, radio equipment, or electronics.

WHAT DOES A BIOMEDICAL EQUIPMENT TECHNICIAN DO?

Biomedical equipment technicians inspect, maintain, repair, and install medical equipment. This equipment includes heart-lung machines, artificial kidney machines, chemical analyzers, magnetic imaging devices, and even artificial hearts. Some technicians assist doctors by operating the equipment as well, even during surgery.

One of the most important jobs biomedical equipment technicians do is fix broken instruments. When a problem arises with equipment, technicians try to find the cause of the problem. If the problem is complicated, technicians might contact the manufacturer of the equipment for help.

Biomedical equipment technicians also install and test new equipment to make sure that it works properly. They often take apart and inspect pieces of equipment. They clean and oil moving parts. They test circuits, meters, and gauges to see that all are operating properly. Technicians also keep records of equipment repairs, maintenance checks, and expenses.

research for their own projects.

Education and Training

To become a biomedical engineer, you will have to earn a college degree. High school science (including biology, chemistry, and physics) and mathematics will be a good basis for study in college. Most biomedical engineers study engineering for four years in a university and then go on for more years of advanced study in biomedical engineering. If you want to direct a research project or teach at the university level you will have to earn a doctorate. The minimum education necessary for any biomedical engineering position is a bachelor's degree.

Biomedical engineers should have a broad interest in the sciences. They have to be able to use their knowledge to solve problems. Often this means working on one problem for a long time and paying attention to every detail of the results. Biomedical engineers also have to be good at working with others because they often work on research teams.

Earnings

The more education biomedical engineers have, the higher their salaries. Biomedical engineers earn between $25,000 and $65,000 a year. Biomedical engineers with doctorates earn the highest salaries.

Salaries increase with experience. Engineers who work for private industry or in hospitals usually earn more than those who work for the government or for universities.

Outlook

As people live longer, the demand for health care will

FOR MORE INFO

For more information about a career in biomedical engineering, contact these organizations:

American Society for Engineering Education
1818 N Street, NW, Suite 600
Washington, DC 20036
Tel: 202-331-3500
Web: http://www.asee.org

Biomedical Engineering Society
PO Box 2399
Culver City, CA 90231
Tel: 310-618-9322
Web: http://mecca.org/BME/BMES/society/index.htm

Canadian Medical and Biological Engineering Society
National Research Council of Canada
Room 393, M-1500
Ottawa, Ontario, K1A 0R8 Canada

increase. This means more jobs for biomedical engineers in the future. As we understand more about how the human body operates, the more work there will be for engineers to help repair and replace body parts that are injured or damaged by disease.

Chiropractors

What Chiropractors Do

Chiropractors are trained primary health care providers, much like physicians. Chiropractors focus on wellness and disease prevention. They look at patients' symptoms. They also consider nutrition, work, stress levels, exercise habits, and posture. Chiropractors treat people of all ages—from children to senior citizens. Doctors of chiropractic most frequently treat conditions such as backache, disc problems, sciatica, and whiplash. They also care for people with headaches, respiratory problems, allergies, digestive trouble, high blood pressure, and many other common ailments. Some specialize in areas such as sports medicine or nutrition. Chiropractors do not use drugs or surgery. If they decide that a patient needs drugs or surgery, they refer the person to another professional.

Doctors of chiropractic look for causes of disorders of the spine. They consider the spine and the nervous system to be

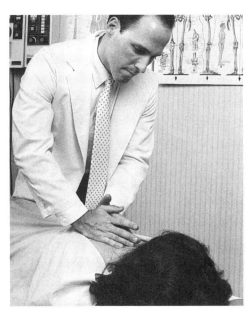

A chiropractor presses along the spine of a patient to adjust the bones.

extremely important to the health of the individual. Chiropractic teaches that problems in the spinal column (backbone) affect the nervous system and the body's natural defense systems. They believe spine problems are the underlying causes of many diseases.

On a patient's first visit, doctors of chiropractic meet with the patient and take a complete medical history before they begin treatment. They ask questions about the person's life to figure out the nature of the illness. Events in the patient's past that may seem unimportant may be very important to the chiropractor. Then chiropractors do a careful physical examination. The examination may include laboratory tests and X rays.

EXPLORING

• Join science clubs.

• Participate in science fairs.

• To develop interviewing and communication skills, you might join the school newspaper staff and ask for interview assignments.

• Learn to play chess or try to solve mystery stories to increase your powers of observation.

• Learn to play an instrument, such as the piano, guitar, or violin, to improve your manual dexterity.

• Learning to give massages is another way to increase manual dexterity.

Once they have made a diagnosis, chiropractic physicians use a variety of ways to help make the person healthy again. The spinal adjustment is the treatment for which chiropractic is most known. During this procedure, patients usually lie on an adjustable table. Chiropractic physicians use their hands to work the spine. They apply pressure and use techniques of manipulation to help the affected areas of the spine. Chiro-

practic treatments must often be repeated over the course of several visits.

In addition to the spinal adjustment, chiropractic physicians may use drugless natural therapies, such as light, water, electrical stimulation, massage, heat, ultrasound, or biofeedback. Chiropractors also make suggestions about diet, rest, and exercise.

Education and Training

To become a doctor of chiropractic, you will have to study a minimum of six to seven years after high school. Most chiropractic colleges require at least two years of undergraduate study before you can enroll. Some require a bachelor's degree.

During the first two years of most chiropractic programs you will spend most of your time in the classroom or the laboratory.

IT'S A FACT

One of the earliest records of chiropractic-type medicine is in the Chinese Kong Fou Document written around 2700 BC. Chiropractic became more recognized about 100 years ago when Daniel David Palmer gave an "adjustment" that was felt to be a misplaced vertebra in the upper spine of a deaf janitor. The janitor then observed that his hearing improved.

Source: American Chiropractic Association

The last two years focus on courses in spinal adjustments. After completing the six- or seven-year program, you will receive the degree of Doctor of Chiropractic (D.C.).

All 50 states and the District of Columbia require chiropractors to obtain a license to practice. Several states require chiropractors to pass a basic science examination as well.

Earnings

The average income for chiropractic physicians is about $228,236 a year. Chiropractors who are employed by someone else have the lowest earnings—about $38,968 a year. Those who work in private practice earn about $84,228 a year. They usually have lower incomes than those in group or partnership, who earn around $102,426 a year.

Outlook

The demand for doctors of chiropractic is expected to grow faster than the average through

FOR MORE INFO

For general information, and a career kit, contact:
American Chiropractic Association
1701 Clarendon Boulevard
Arlington, VA 22209
Tel: 800-986-4636
Web: http://www.amerchiro.org

For information on educational requirements and accredited colleges, contact:
Council on Chiropractic Education
7975 North Hayden Road, Suite A-210
Scottsdale, AZ 85258
Tel: 602-443-8877

For information on student membership, contact:
International Chiropractors Association
1110 North Glebe Road, Suite 1000
Arlington, VA 22201
Tel: 800-423-4690
Web: http//www.chiropractic.org

2006. Many areas have a shortage of chiropractors. More insurance policies and HMOs now cover chiropractic services. While the demand for chiropractic is increasing, college enrollments are also growing. New chiropractors may find increasing competition for jobs.

Dental Hygienists

The Way It Was

The first dental hygienists were trained by dentists themselves. Early in the 20th century, the first school for dental hygiene was started, and in 1915, the first state legalized the practice of dental hygiene.

RELATED JOBS

Dental Assistants
Dental Laboratory Technicians
Dentists

What Dental Hygienists Do

Dental hygienists work for dentists. They are licensed to clean patients' teeth. Their main job is to remove plaque and other deposits from the teeth, polish teeth, and massage gums. They also teach good oral health. They show patients how to select toothbrushes and use floss, what kinds of foods damage the teeth, and the effects of habits, such as smoking, on teeth. The main goal of a dental hygienist is to help patients prevent tooth and gum decay and keep a healthy mouth.

Hygienists who work for dentists in private practice may do more than clean teeth. They may take and develop X rays, mix materials to fill cavities, sterilize instruments, assist in surgery, and keep charts of patients' teeth. Some hygienists have office duties as well, such as answering phone calls and making appointments for patients.

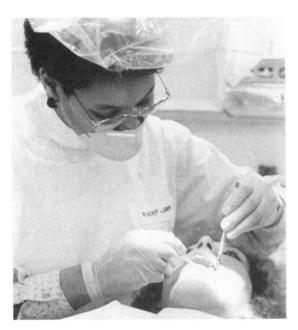

A dental hygienist cleans a patient's teeth.

Not all hygienists work for dentists. Some work in schools where they clean and examine students' teeth and show them how to prevent tooth decay. They teach children and teens how to brush and floss teeth correctly and eat the right foods. They also keep records of the students' teeth and tell parents about any problems or need for more treatment.

Some dental hygienists work for local, state, or federal public health agencies. They clean the teeth of adults and children in public health clinics and other public facilities and educate patients in the proper care of teeth.

EXPLORING

• Ask your dental hygienist to show you the tools he or she uses. Hygienists will be happy to answer any questions you may have about their jobs.

• Learn about dental care. Practice good dental hygiene.

Education and Training

To become a dental hygienist, you must

WHAT DO DENTAL LABORATORY TECHNICIANS DO?

You may never see a *dental laboratory technician* in your dentist's office, but they are very important in many different kinds of dental treatment. When someone loses a tooth, for example, the dentist writes a prescription for a new one and the technician makes it in a laboratory.

Some technicians make braces for straightening teeth by bending wires into complicated shapes that will fit over the crooked teeth. The braces, retainers, or tooth bands that these technicians make are not permanent, but will stay in a patient's mouth for a long time, so they must fit well and feel comfortable.

Dental ceramicists make real-looking porcelain teeth to replace missing ones or to fit over natural teeth that may have been damaged. Ceramicists apply porcelain paste over a metal frame to make crowns, bridges, and tooth coverings.

Some dental laboratory technicians make and repair full and partial dentures. Full dentures are false teeth worn by people who have had all their teeth removed on the upper or lower jaws or on both jaws. Partial dentures are the missing teeth that are placed in a jaw alongside the natural teeth. Dentures are made by putting ceramic teeth in a wax model and then building up wax over it to hold the set in place.

Crown and bridge specialists make the missing parts of a natural tooth that has broken. They use plastic and metal parts that are permanently cemented to the natural tooth. These technicians must be skilled at melting and casting metals.

have a high school diploma. Then you must complete two or four years of college at an accredited dental hygiene school, and pass the national board exams for your state.

There are two types of dental hygiene programs. One is a four-year college program offering a bachelor's degree. The other is a two-year program leading to a dental hygiene certification. More employers now require a four-year degree. During your education, you will study anatomy, physiology, chemistry, pharmacology, nutrition, and other sciences. You will also learn to handle delicate instruments, gain experience in the dental laboratory, and practice working with patients in clinics.

Earnings

Hygienists who work in private dentists' offices earn higher incomes than those working in school systems, public health agencies, hospitals, factories, or the armed forces.

According to the U.S. Department of Labor, full-time dental hygienists earn between $24,000 and $39,500 a year. Beginning hygienists earn an average of $15,200 to $17,500 a year. Salaries in large cities are generally higher than in smaller cities and towns.

Outlook

Employment opportunities for dental hygienists are promising

FOR MORE INFO

For publications, information on dental schools, and scholarship information, contact:
American Association of Dental Schools
1625 Massachusetts Avenue, NW
Suite 600
Washington, DC 20036
Tel: 202-667-9433
Email: aads@aads.jhu.edu
Web: http://www.aads.jhu.edu

For education information, contact:
American Dental Association
211 East Chicago Avenue
Chicago, IL 60611
Tel: 312-440-2500
Web: http://www.ada.org/prac/careers/apl-03.html

For career information and tips for dental hygiene students on finding a job, contact:
American Dental Hygienists' Association
444 North Michigan Avenue, Suite 3400
Chicago, IL 60611
Tel: 312-440-8900
Email: mail@adha.net
Web: http://www.adha.org

through 2006. As the population increases and more employers offer dental insurance, there will be more jobs for dental hygienists.

Dentists

What Dentists Do

Dentists help people have healthy teeth and gums. They do this by cleaning, filling, repairing, replacing, and straightening teeth. Dentists who are general practitioners do many kinds of dental work. They take X rays, fill cavities, clean teeth, and pull diseased teeth. Dentists also talk to their patients about how they can prevent tooth and mouth problems. They give patients instructions on proper brushing, flossing, and diet. They must also be able to recognize problems that need the care of a dental specialist.

Orthodontists are dental specialists who use braces and other devices to correct irregular growth of teeth and jaws. *Oral surgeons* perform difficult tooth-pulling jobs. They remove tumors and fix broken jaws. *Periodontists* treat diseased gums. *Prosthodontists* make artificial teeth and dentures. *Pedodontists* treat children's dental problems. *Oral pathologists* examine mouth tumors and sores and deter-

What Causes Bad Breath?

There are lots of reasons why people have bad breath:
• The foods you eat can affect the air you exhale—onions and garlic, for instance. The odor will stay in your breath until your body finishes processing the food.
• If you don't brush your teeth and floss every day, the food particles in your mouth collect bacteria. That bacteria causes bad odors.
• Periodontal (gum) disease can cause bad breath. Periodontal disease happens when the plaque builds up on your teeth and irritates your gums.
• Smoking not only causes bad breath, but it can stain your teeth and also lead to periodontal disease or oral cancer.
• Bad breath may be a sign of a medical problem somewhere else in your body. For example, a respiratory infection, bronchitis, diabetes, and liver or kidney disease can all cause bad breath.

mine their cause. *Endodontists* treat patients who need root canals.

About 90 percent of dentists have their own private practices. Because dentists work for themselves, they have to know about business matters, such as leasing office space, hiring employees, running an office, keeping books, and stocking equipment. Most dentists work at least 40 hours a week, including some time on weekends.

Education and Training

In high school, science and math courses are a good preparation for a career in dentistry. To become a dentist, you must complete three to four years of college-level predental education. Three out of four dentists have a bachelor's or master's degree. After college, you must go to a certified dental school. Then you must pass the Dental Admissions Test. Training at a dental school then takes at least four years. During this time, you will study basic sciences, including anatomy, biochemistry, microbiology, and physiology, as well as how to treat patients. After graduation, a dentist must take a state examination to receive a license to practice dentistry. Dentists who wish to enter a specialized field spend an additional

EXPLORING

• There are lots of hobbies that will develop strength and agility in your fingers and hands. Try sculpting, metalworking, model making, fine needlework, or any other activity where you need to do precise work with tiny parts.

• Learn all you can about dental care and practice good dental hygiene:

1. Eat a balanced diet. Limit the snacks you eat, especially ones that contain sugar and starch. If you must snack, eat cheese, raw vegetables, plain yogurt, or fruit.

2. Brush your teeth twice a day with a fluoride toothpaste.

3. Floss between your teeth every day.

WHAT DO ORTHODONTISTS DO?

Orthodontists are dentists who have special training in the diagnosis, prevention, and treatment of dental and facial problems. The technical term for these types of problems is "malocclusion," which means "bad bite." Orthodontists design and apply corrective appliances, such as braces, which slowly move patients' teeth, lips, and jaws into proper alignment. Extremely severe alignment problems may require orthodontists to perform surgery.

Orthodontists take X rays and photographs of the teeth that need to be adjusted. Then they make models of the patients' teeth and jaws to evaluate patients' dental and skeletal conditions. After they examine patients' mouths, orthodontists prescribe either fixed or removable braces. Patients return to their orthodontists periodically throughout their treatment to have their braces or other corrective appliances adjusted. As patients progress through treatment, orthodontists make sure that teeth are moving correctly and that jaws are developing properly. After braces are removed, orthodontists work with patients to make sure that teeth stay in their new positions.

Although orthodontists treat people of all ages, the majority of patients are teenagers. Most teens treated by orthodontists have to wear braces for one to three years. Some adults also see orthodontists to reduce tooth loss from periodontal (gum) disease, to treat symptoms of temporomandibular joint (TMJ) dysfunction, and to improve the appearance of teeth and jaws.

Education and Training: After graduation from dental school and getting your license, you must complete a two- to three-year program leading to a certificate or a master's degree in orthodontics.

Earnings: The average income of all dental specialists, including orthodontists, is about $197,000 a year.

Outlook: The employment outlook for orthodontists is good through 2006.

two to three years studying that specialty.

Earnings

Opening a dental office is expensive. Dentists who are beginning a private practice often earn only enough to pay their expenses. Some dentists start by working for an established dentist until they can earn their own reputation and save enough money to equip an office. According to the American Dental Association, the average income of self-employed dentists is about $120,000 a year. Specialists average $192,000 a year.

Outlook

Opportunities for dentists are expected to grow more slowly than the average through 2006. There will be more jobs, though, for dental specialists. Cosmetic dentists, oral pathologists and orthodontists, for instance, will be in great demand.

FOR MORE INFO

For information on admission requirements of U.S. and Canadian dental schools, contact:
American Association of Dental Schools
1625 Massachusetts Avenue, NW, Suite 600
Washington, DC 20036
Tel: 202-667-9433
Email: aads@aads.jhu.edu
Web: http://www.aads.jhu.edu/

For a list of accredited schools for postgraduate and postdoctoral work, contact:
American Dental Association
Department of Career Guidance
211 East Chicago Avenue
Chicago, IL 60611
Tel: 312-440-2500
Web: http://www.ada.org/tc-educ.html

For information on careers in dentistry, visit this Web site:
So you want to be a dentist?
Web: http://www.vvm.com/
~bond/home.htm

RELATED JOBS

Dental Assistants
Dental Hygienists
Dental Laboratory Technicians
Endodontists
Orthodontists
Periodontists
Physicians

Emergency Medical Technicians

What Emergency Medical Technicians Do

Emergency medical technicians, or *EMTs,* drive in ambulances or fly in helicopters to the scene of accidents or emergencies to care for ill or injured people.

EMTs decide what kind of medical help victims need and treat them quickly. They may set broken bones or try to restart someone's heart. They must be able to stay calm and to calm others in a crisis.

The ambulances and helicopters EMTs use have two-way radios. At the scene of an emergency, EMTs may need to make radio contact with hospitals to ask for a physician's advice about treatment. On the way to the hospital, EMTs radio ahead so the emergency room is ready. They help carry the victims into the hospital, and give the hospital staff as much information as they can about the patient's condition and the nature of the accident. EMTs must keep their ambulances and helicopters in good order and make sure that they always have the equipment they need.

EMTs work for hospitals, fire departments, police departments, private ambulance services, or other first-aid organizations. In fire departments, some EMTs work 56 hours a week. Most others work 40 hours a week. Since people need emergency help at all hours, EMTs work nights, weekends, and holidays.

Education and Training

To be an EMT, you must first finish high school. You have to be at least 18 years old, and have a driver's license. High school courses in health, physics, chemistry, and mathematics are helpful. A course in driver's education will be useful because EMTs need excellent driving skills. You need to know the roads and travel conditions in your area so you can drive to the scene of an emergency and to the hospital quickly and safely.

Many hospitals, colleges, and police and fire departments offer the basic EMT training course. The federal government requires all EMTs to pass this basic training course, which teaches you how to deal with common medical emergencies.

EXPLORING

• You may be able to take a first aid class or training in cardiopulmonary resuscitation. Organizations such as the Red Cross or a nearby hospital can provide information on local training courses.

• When you get to high school, you may be able to volunteer at hospitals or clinics to learn more about medicine and health care.

Amkus cutter: A hand-held rescue device, similar to scissors, used to free trapped victims by cutting through metal.

Amkus rams: A hand-held rescue device used to free trapped victims by pushing or pulling obstructions, such as dashboard and seats, away from the victim.

Amkus spreader: A hand-held rescue device used to free trapped victims by pulling crumpled metal apart.

Backboard: A long, flat, hard surface used to immobilize the spine in case of neck or spinal injury.

Defibrillator: A machine with electrodes to apply electric currents to heart muscles in order to shock the muscles into operation.

Endotracheal intubation: The insertion of a tube into the trachea, or windpipe, to provide a passage for air, in case of obstruction.

The National Registry of Emergency Medical Technicians (NREMT) sets standards for EMTs across the country. To be listed on this registry, EMTs must finish the basic training program, have six months work experience, and pass both a written and a practical test to prove they can handle medical emergencies.

All states require EMTs to earn state certification by passing a state exam or fulfilling the basic NREMT registration requirements.

Earnings

EMTs who work in the public sector for police and fire departments usually receive a higher wage than those who work for ambulance companies and hospitals. Average pay for an experienced EMT-basic in a private ambulance service is $19,383 a year. Those who work in fire departments earn about $31,141 a year. Those classified as EMT-basic earn about $22,848 a year. Those who are EMT-I (intermediate) earn $24,682 a year. EMT-paramedics earn $28,079 a year.

Outlook

The outlook for EMTs should remain good in larger communities. In smaller communities with fewer financial resources, the outlook for employment may stay limited. The growing number of older people in the United States, who use emergency medical services more often than others, should increase the need for EMTs.

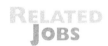

RELATED
JOBS

Firefighters
Medical Assistants
Nurses
Physician Assistants
Physicians
Surgical Technologists

FOR MORE INFO

This organization represents companies that provide emergency and nonemergency medical transportation services:
American Ambulance Association
1255 23rd Street, NW
Washington, DC 20037-1174
Tel: 202-452-8888
Email: aaa911@the-aaa.org
Web: http://www.the-aaa.org

For information on EMT careers, contact:
National Association of Emergency Medical Technicians
102 West Leake Street
Clinton, MS 39056
Tel: 800-346-2368

For information on testing for EMT certification, contact:
National Registry of Emergency Medical Technicians
PO Box 29233
6610 Busch Boulevard
Columbus, OH 43229
Tel: 614-888-4484
Web: http://www.nremt.org

Fitness Experts

What Fitness Experts Do

Fitness experts teach people how to exercise, eat right, and have a healthy lifestyle. Everyone has different fitness needs, so experts must design programs specially for each person's needs. Even when they teach classes, they must plan programs that will meet the needs of people at different levels of health and fitness.

Aerobics instructors teach aerobic dance and aerobic step classes. They sometimes teach special groups, such as the elderly or those with injuries or illnesses that affect their ability to exercise. They also teach those without health problems who just want to be fit and stay healthy. Aerobics instructors use lively exercise routines set to music that can be changed to fit the needs of each individual class.

The term aerobic refers to the body's need for oxygen during the exercise. Aerobic exercise strengthens the heart and cardiovascular (blood) system. A typical class starts with warm-up exercises, or slow stretching movements that get the blood moving and increase flexibility. After the warm-up are about 30 minutes of non-stop activity to increase the heart rate. The class ends with a cool-down period of stretching and slower movements.

Aerobics instructors teach at almost every type of club or community group, including community centers, churches, YMCA or YWCAs, health clubs, and park or recreation districts. Businesses may also hire an instructor to teach classes for their employees.

Personal trainers, often called *fitness trainers,* help health-conscious people with exercise, weight training, weight loss, diet and nutrition, and medical reha-bilitation programs. During one training session, or over a period of several ses-sions, trainers teach their clients how to achieve their health and fitness goals. They may train in the homes of their clients, their own studio spaces, or in health clubs. Approximately 55,000 per-sonal trainers work in the United States.

Education and Training

If you're interested in health and fitness, you are probably already taking physical

EXPLORING

• Visit a health club, park district, or YMCA aerobics class to observe the work of fit-ness trainers and aero-bics instructors.

• Enroll in an aerobics class or train with a fit-ness trainer to experi-ence firsthand what their jobs are like.

• Participate in school sports.

• Join local athletic clubs or start one your-self. Get a group of friends together to run or ride bikes at a regu-lar time each week. Measure your fitness progress.

• Learn about nutrition and practice good dietary habits.

education classes and involved in sports activities. It's also important to take health courses and courses like home economics, which include lessons in diet and nutrition. Business courses can help you if you plan to run your own personal training service. Science courses such as biology, chemistry, and physiology are important for your understanding of muscle groups, food and drug reactions, and other concerns of exercise science.

Most fitness instructors have a high school diploma and many now have college degrees. A college major in either sports physiology or exercise physiology will help if you want to advance to health club director or teach wellness programs.

Aerobics instructors are often required to become certified by an organization, such as the American Council on Exercise. Certification usually involves passing a written exam. To pass the exam, you will need to know how medications affect the body, how nutrition affects performance, how to teach special groups, and how to handle injuries in class. Aerobics instructors also must be certified in CPR.

Workshops are taught usually in adult education courses at such places as the YMCA, to help you gain experience. Unpaid apprenticeships are a good way to get supervised experience before you teach classes on your own.

A college education isn't required to work as a personal trainer, but you can benefit from one of the many fitness-related programs offered at colleges across the country. Some relevant college programs are: health education, exercise and sports science, fitness program management, and athletic training.

Earnings

Instructors are usually paid by the class, and usually start out at about $10 per class. Experienced aerobics instructors can earn up to $50 or $60 per class. Health club directors usually earn about $30,000 a year.

Over one-half of personal trainers earn an hourly wage of about $20 to $30 or more. Average yearly salaries range from $20,000 to $40,000 and more. Most independent contractors are paid by the hour. The top three factors that determine pay are certification, continuing education, and years in the industry.

Outlook

Because of the country's increasing interest in overall health and fitness, the job outlook for fitness experts should remain strong in the next decade. As the population continues to age, many aerobics instructors will be needed to work in retirement homes as

FOR MORE INFO

For information about personal fitness trainer certification, contact:
National Athletic Trainers' Association
2952 Stemmons Freeway, Suite 200
Dallas, TX 75247-6916
Tel: 214-637-6282, ext. 108
Email: suzannec@nata.org
Web: http://www.nata.org

For more information about careers in fitness, contact:
American Council on Exercise
5820 Oberlin Drive, Suite 102
San Diego, CA 92121-3787
Tel: 619-535-8227
Web: http://www.acefitness.org

For information about the fitness industry in general, and personal training specifically, contact:
IDEA Health and Fitness Source
6190 Cornerstone Court East, Suite 204
San Diego, CA 92121-3773
Tel: 800-999-4332, ext. 7
Email: member@ideafit.com
Web: http://www.ideafit.com

well. Many large businesses will also hire instructors to help keep their employees healthy and their health insurance costs down.

Health Care Managers

Where Do Health Care Managers Work?

There were about 320,000 health care managers in the 1990s. More than half of them worked in hospitals. Health care managers also work in:

Medical group practices

Long-term care facilities

Nursing homes

Rehabilitation institutions

Psychiatric hospitals

Health maintenance organizations (HMOs)

Outpatient clinics

What Health Care Managers Do

Health care managers direct the operation of health care organizations. These include hospitals, nursing homes, medical group practices, long-term care facilities, rehabilitation clinics, and health maintenance organizations (HMOs). They are responsible for the building, equipment, services, staff, budgets, and relations with other organizations.

Health care managers organize and manage a wide variety of activities. They hire and supervise employees, figure budgets, set fees to be charged to patients, and establish billing methods. They buy supplies and equipment and set up ways to maintain the building and equipment. They make sure there are mail, phone, and laundry services for patients and staff. They make sure that their facility meets certain standards. Together with the medical staff and department heads, they develop training programs for staff.

Health care managers work closely with their facility's board of directors to develop plans and policies. Health care managers may also carry out large projects, such as fund-raising campaigns that help the facility change, update, and develop its services.

Education and Training

To prepare for this career, you should begin in high school by taking classes in mathematics, computer science, health, biology, chemistry, and social studies. After high school, you should go to college and take a wide range of courses, such as social sciences, economics, and business administration.

Many health care facilities hire only managers who have master's degrees in hospital or health services administration or a similar field. Some places hire managers who are physicians or registered nurses, or have training in law or business along with health care experience.

Earnings

Salaries of health care managers depend on the type of facility, location, the size of the staff, and the budget. Average salaries of hospital managers is about $190,500 a year. Nursing home administrators earn

EXPLORING

• Health care managers need to be leaders and talented speakers. To learn these skills you can participate in clubs of any kind as a leader or member. Join debate and speech clubs to develop speaking skills.

• When you get a little older, you can volunteer to work in a hospital or nursing home. This can help you learn about how health care facilities operate.

How It All Began

The Pennsylvania Hospital was established in Philadelphia in the mid-1700s by Benjamin Franklin and Dr. Thomas Bond. Since then, health care institutions have changed considerably. For example, medical science has advanced rapidly and physicians have become highly specialized. Complicated equipment has been invented, creating a need for technicians. With this growth rose a need for health care managers to organize and supervise operations.

Hospital administration as a separate profession began in the 1890s when the Association of Hospital Superintendents was organized. Today, nearly all of the hospitals in the United States belong to this group, which is now known as the American Hospital Association. In the 1930s the American College of Hospital Administrators (now the American College of Healthcare Executives) was started to raise the standards of practice and education in the field.

It's a Fact

The field of long-term care is one of the fastest growing parts of the health care industry. Today, there are over 15,000 nursing homes in the United States.

about $49,500 a year. Assistant nursing home administrators earn salaries of $32,000 a year.

Health services administrators who manage a small group have average salaries of $56,000 a year. Administrators who manage medical practices with more than seven physicians earn an average of $77,000 a year.

Outlook

Employment in health care will be excellent through 2006. The number of hospitals is declining, but separate companies are being started to provide services such as outpatient surgery, alcohol and drug rehabilitation, or home health care. Many new openings should be available in settings other than hospitals.

With hospitals trying to lower costs and increase earnings, demand for business school graduates should remain steady.

For More Info

For more information about a career as a health care manager, contact:

American College of Health Care Administrators
325 South Patrick Street
Alexandria, VA 22314-3571
Tel: 703-549-5822
Web: http://www.achca.org

American College of Healthcare Executives
One North Franklin Street, Suite 1700
Chicago, IL 60606-3491
Tel: 312-424-2800
Web: http://www.ache.org

Healthcare Financial Management Association
2 Westbrook Corporate Center, Suite 700
Westchester, IL 60154-5700
Tel: 800-252-HFMA
Web: http://www.hfma.org

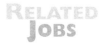

Related Jobs

Business Managers
City Managers
Physicians

Home Health Care Aides

What Home Health Care Aides Do

Home health care aides care for people who live at home but are unable to care for themselves. Home health care aides usually assist the elderly or people with disabilities. They also work with children of parents with disabilities and people who are sick and need help for a short period of time. Aides help with such day-to-day tasks as laundry, shopping, and cooking. This assistance allows many people to stay at home instead of having to stay in nursing homes or other health care facilities. Job duties vary with the client's needs. For example, a home health care aide may help a client out of bed and into a wheelchair or change the clothes of patients who cannot do it by themselves. Aides often bathe clients, help with household chores, and prepare meals. For clients who have suffered an injury or are ill, home health care aides may help them do exercises, check vital signs (pulse, blood pressure, and temper-

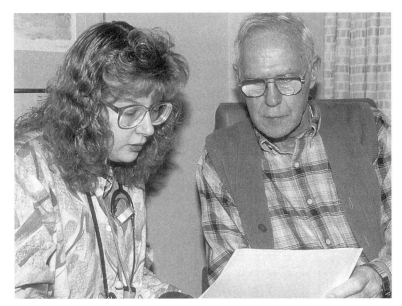

A home health care aide explains a new sugar-free diet plan to one of her clients.

ature), or assist with medications. Home health care aides may also give bedridden people massages to keep their muscles strong. All of these health-related tasks are directed by a physician or registered nurse.

Home health care aides also provide emotional support. The aide may be the only person a client sees for long periods of time. The aide may cheer the person up and perhaps listen and give advice on personal problems. Often, an aide plays cards or other types of games with a client to keep the client occupied during the long hours at home.

Responsibilities vary and so does the length of time a home health care aide

EXPLORING

• **Contact local agencies and programs that provide home care services and request information on their employment guidelines or training programs.**
• **Help a parent or older sister or brother care for an elderly relative or neighbor. You might offer to play cards or other games. You could help do the laundry or cook a meal.**
• **Many communities have adopt-a-grandparent programs for children and teens.**

THE BEGINNINGS OF HOME HEALTH CARE

A typical household back in the 1800s often included an elderly parent or ill or injured relative. Families didn't have many of the modern conveniences we have today, so regular household chores could be impossible for someone weakened by illness or age. It was common for parents to move in with their grown children when they became unable to look after themselves. The needs of the elderly or sick person often took far more time and energy than the family could give. Running a household left little time for the family to care for the seriously ill.

Rural areas began to make "visiting nurses" available to check on patients who lived far from town and had no way to travel to doctor's offices. These nurses found that the needs of the patients went beyond medical care. Patients were thankful for the company of another person in their homes, someone to read their mail to them or run errands. The demand for this kind of home care increased and the profession of home care aides began to grow.

Advances in modern medicine have made it possible for many illnesses to be treated at home. The medical profession is also recognizing that people usually recover from illnesses better when they are treated in their homes.

works with a client. Aides may help someone just released from the hospital on a daily basis for a few weeks or they may help an elderly person several times a week for an indefinite period.

Education and Training

There are no specific educational requirements for jobs in this field. Most employers prefer to hire those with a high school diploma and some experience working with the sick or elderly. Volunteer work with sick and/or elderly people also is good experience. Many agencies provide several weeks of training to teach new aides how to bathe and care for patients and how to do basic housekeeping and cooking tasks.

Home health care aides do not have to pass any tests or be licensed to work. But if a client's services are paid by Medicare, you need special training programs and you must be certified.

Earnings

Working hours and patient loads vary quite a bit. For many aides who begin as part-time employees, the starting salary usually is the minimum hourly wage ($5). For full-time aides with training or experience, earnings may be around $6 to $8 an hour.

Outlook

Government and private agencies are developing more programs to assist the elderly and people with disabilities. This means that the need for home health care aides will continue to grow. The number of people 70 years of age and older should increase in the next ten

FOR MORE INFO

For information about a career as a home health care aide and schools offering training, contact:
National Association for Home Care
228 Seventh Street, SE
Washington, DC 20003
Tel: 202-547-7424
Web: http://www.nahc.org

National Association of Health Career Schools
750 First Street, NE, Suite 940
Washington, DC 20002
Email: NAHCS@aol.com

years. Many of them will need at least some home care. Because of the work of home health care aides, hospitals and nursing homes can offer quality care to more people. This job is very demanding, both physically and emotionally, so aides frequently change jobs and find other careers. This means that there are always job openings for home health care aides.

Hospice Workers

What Hospice Workers Do

Hospice is a special kind of care for patients in the last stage of a terminal illness. *Hospice workers* include a wide variety of specially trained health care professionals. They help these patients live comfortably in their last days or weeks of life.

Traditional medicine focuses on treating and healing patients. Hospice programs try to improve dying patients' lives when treatments no longer work. Hospices view dying as a normal process, and the illness is allowed to run its course. Some hospice patients improve and leave the program to resume medical treatment.

Hospice programs are found in hospitals, private care facilities, and in the homes of patients. Hospice workers help patients with terminal illnesses, such as cancer, AIDS, Alzheimer's, or Parkinson's. Patients have a range of health conditions. Some are bedridden, while some can still take care of themselves.

Hospice medical directors are physicians who oversee the medical program and advise the hospice care staff. *Field supervisors, supervisors of home health care aides,* and *supervisors of rehabilitation services* oversee the activities of their hospice teams. They make sure each patient is properly cared for by the various hospice specialists.

Registered nurses visit patients regularly to monitor their emotional and physical symptoms. *Nurse assistants* and *home health care aides* help the family with the personal care of the patient. They bathe, groom, and change the bed linen of their patients.

Physical therapists, occupational therapists, and *speech therapists* help patients with daily living tasks that have become difficult or impossible to perform. They may help patients to walk, dress, or feed themselves, or help those who have lost their ability to speak.

Social workers help patients and families emotionally. They may simply be good listeners who try to relieve any fears or

EXPLORING

• You may be able to volunteer to visit the sick to cheer them up or help with small chores. Your school, church, or a community organization may have such a program.

• Offer to help care for sick relatives or neighbors. You can run errands, do light chores, or just spend time with them. Read to them, play card games or board games, or just chat.

ADVICE FOR HOSPICE WORKERS: MAKE 'EM LAUGH!

In 1976, the famous writer and editor, Norman Cousins, wrote an article for the New England Journal of Medicine. He described his experience with a severe kind of arthritis. This illness causes pain, fatigue, heart problems, and lung disease. The joints swell and stiffen up and the spine becomes rigid. Cousins decided to fight his illness with laughter. He told jokes and listened to them. He watched silly movies and began to realize that the more he laughed, the less pain he felt. He says he was eventually "cured" by regular doses of laughter.

There have been many studies on the effect of laughter on illness. These studies show the following:

• Happy people are less likely to develop cancer than unhappy people.
• Laughter, joy, and happiness boost the immune system's ability to fight viruses and infection.
• Soothing music can help the body withstand pain better.

worries that patients or families may have. They may also help them find personal and community support. *Chaplains* provide religious support to patients and families. *Music therapists* use music to provide comfort and relaxation to patients. They often sing or play a musical instrument for their patients or play recorded selections.

Grief therapists help the family after the patient has died. Their services are usually available for up to one year after the family member has passed away.

Education and Training

The educational requirements for hospice workers vary greatly. Nurse assistants and home health care aides need very little training after high school. Physicians, though, need six to nine years of education after college.

There are only a few colleges and universities that offer specialized hospice degrees. Many hospitals offer medical training in hospice care to physicians, nurses, and other professionals.

Earnings

Salaries for hospice workers are similar to what they would earn in other places, such as hospitals and nursing homes. The median national salary for hospice directors is $52,500 a year. (See the chapters in this book on *Nurses, Nurse Assistants, Home Health Care Aides, Physicians* and *Physical Therapists*.)

Outlook

Hospice workers will be needed to take care of the growing number of elderly people. Cancer patients will also continue to need care. Many patients choose hospice programs because they cost less than long-term hospital care. More health care professionals and

FOR MORE INFO

For more information on careers in hospice programs, contact:

Hospice Education Institute
190 Westbrook Road
Essex, CT 06426
Tel: 203-767-1620

Hospice Association of America
228 Seventh Street, SE
Washington, DC 20003-4306
Web: http://www.nahc.org

patients choose hospice because of its spiritual, patient-centered focus.

RELATED JOBS

Advanced Practice Nurses
HIV/AIDS Counselors
Grief Therapists
Home Health Care Aides
Nurse Assistants
Nurses
Physicians
Social Workers

Medical Record Technicians

What Medical Record Technicians Do

Any hospital, clinic, or physician's office keeps detailed records on patients. These records tell what injuries or illnesses patients have been treated for and how well they've responded to treatment. *Medical record technicians* are in charge of putting together, organizing, and storing the medical records for all the patients who are treated in a hospital or in a physician's office. They use filing systems to keep track of this information.

Medical records are very complicated. All records show the patient's medical history, the results of physical examinations, and notes on any hospital stays. They list medications that have been prescribed, and any side effects the patient experienced. This information is later used by doctors, insurance companies, researchers, and others. For example, someone may need to see records of all babies born in the hospital in the past five years. Medical record technicians make sure this information is easy to find and well indexed. They might also create reports, using certain information from a large number of patient records.

All the information in the records is coded using a standard coding system. This system gives numbers to every disease, condition, and procedure. Using a code manual, medical record technicians enter this information into the filing system. Because the same code system is used by all health care professionals, a patient's medical records can be easily reviewed by caregivers across the country. Most medical facilities use computers to index medical records.

Most medical record technicians work in hospitals. Some work in nursing homes, clinics, and doctors' offices. Others work for insurance companies or public health departments.

Education and Training

Classes in English, mathematics, and biology help you prepare for this career. Medical record technicians need a two-year college degree. There are several colleges and schools throughout the United States that offer these degrees.

EXPLORING

• Volunteer to be the secretary or treasurer for any clubs you belong to. These jobs will train you to keep careful notes and organize details.

• When you get to high school, you may be able to find summer, part-time, or volunteer work in a hospital or other health care facility. Sometimes such jobs are available in the medical records department for volunteers who can type or have clerical experience.

You can also become a technician by taking a home study course offered by the American Health Information Management Association (AHIMA), along with 30 credit hours in related courses at a college.

Medical record science includes both classroom study and practical training, such as how to put statistics together or the different ways hospital departments keep records. There are also courses in ethics, since you must know when and how to give out information without violating the patient's right to privacy.

Many medical record technicians choose to become registered with AHIMA. To be registered, you must pass an examination and become an Accredited Record Technician (ART).

WORDS TO LEARN

Transcribing: Making written copies of orally dictated material.

Coding: In medical records, assigning numbers for systematic classification.

Stat: Immediately.

DRG (Diagnosis-Related Grouping): A system used by Medicare and many insurance companies to classify medical patients' care and treatment.

Terminal Digit Order: A numerical filing method emphasizing the last two digits, which is the most effective use of filing space, as well as the most effective method to ensure patient privacy.

ICD (International Classification of Diseases): The numerical classification system used to code diagnoses.

CPT (Common Procedural Terminology): The numerical classification system used in the medical records field to code procedures and treatments.

Source-oriented chart order: A system of organizing patient charts by grouping information into sections based on different health care departments, such as nursing, radiology, or attending physician.

Earnings

Starting salaries for accredited medical record technicians are between $20,000 and $25,000 per year. Experienced technicians in managerial positions can earn up to $48,000 a year. A medical records technician with a bachelor's or other advanced degree can earn $50,000 to $80,000 a year.

Outlook

The Bureau of Labor Statistics says health information technology is one of the 20 fastest growing occupations in the United States. There should be many openings in the medical records field through the next decade, as the medical and insurance industries grow. Medical record technicians will be needed to manage the records and results of sophisticated machinery and diagnostic procedures.

FOR MORE INFO

For information on careers in health information management and ART accreditation, contact:

American Health Information Management Association
919 North Michigan Avenue, Suite 1400
Chicago, IL 60611
Tel: 312-787-2672
Web: http://www.ahima.org

For a list of schools offering accredited programs in health information management, contact:

Commission on Accreditation of Allied Health Education Programs
American Medical Association
35 E. Wacker Drive, Suite 1970
Chicago, IL 60601-2200
Tel: 312-464-5000
Web: http://www.cahep.org

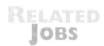

RELATED JOBS

Clerks
Library Technicians
Medical Assistants
Secretaries

Medical Secretaries

What Medical Secretaries Do

Medical secretaries do the administrative and clerical work in medical offices, hospitals, or private doctors' offices. They keep records, answer phone calls, order supplies, handle correspondence, bill patients, complete insurance forms, and transcribe dictation. Medical secretaries also keep financial records and handle other bookkeeping. They greet patients, make appointments, obtain medical histories, arrange hospital admissions, and schedule surgeries.

Medical secretaries play important roles in the healthcare profession. They help physicians or medical scientists with reports, speeches, articles, and conference proceedings. Most medical secretaries need to be familiar with insurance rules, billing practices, and hospital or laboratory procedures.

Doctors rely on medical secretaries to

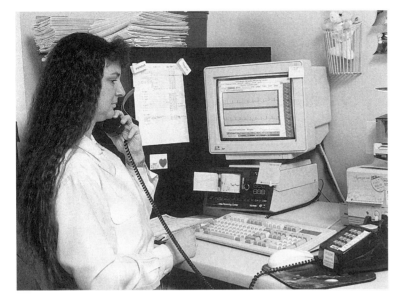

control administrative operations. They spend a lot of time on the phone scheduling appointments and giving information to callers. They organize and maintain paper and computer files, and handle correspondence for themselves and others. They might also type letters and handle travel arrangements. Medical secretaries operate fax machines and photocopiers. They use computers to run spreadsheet, word-processing, database-management, and desktop publishing programs.

Medical secretaries play a major role in large health organizations, such as clinical, research, and educational programs. Medical secretaries also are hired to fill positions as radiology and surgical recorders and medical transcriptionists.

EXPLORING

• Volunteer to be the secretary for any clubs you belong to.
• Offer to be the secretary for your class or run for a student government secretary position.
• Ask your school guidance counselor to set up an information interview with a medical secretary, or arrange a tour of a medical facility so you can see medical secretaries in action.

Education and Training

Most employers require medical secretaries to have high school diplomas or the equivalent. You must be able to type between 60 and 90 words per minute. You must know medical terms and office procedures. You must be familiar with computers and be able to use medical software programs. Good writing, speak-ing, and basic math skills are important.

Some community colleges and vocational schools offer medical secretarial training, including medical stenography, comput-ers, typing, accounting, filing, first aid, medical terminology, and medical office procedures.

Medical secretaries must use

WHERE DID THE WORD "SECRETARY" COME FROM?

The word secretary comes from the same Latin word that gave us secret, according to "The History of the Secretarial Profession" from the International Association of Administrative Professionals. Originally, it meant, "one entrusted with the secrets and confidences of a superior." Probably the ear-liest use of the word was in relation to those people who per-formed jobs for a king. Kings usually would have their trusted agents handle correspondence on private or secret matters.

In 1847, the first Merriam-Webster dictionary defined secre-tary as "a person employed by a public body, or by a company or by an individual, to write orders, letters, dispatches, public or pri-vate papers, records, and the like." Today, secretaries are some-times called administrative professionals.

good judgment in dealing with private medical records. You must be confident when talking to people, both in person and on the telephone. You need a pleasant personality and a desire to help others.

Earnings

Starting salaries for medical secretaries are about $24,000 a year. With some experience, they earn about $29,900 a year. Some medical secretaries earn as much as $35,500 yearly.

Outlook

Growth of the health care field will mean faster than average employment growth for medical secretaries. Organizations are demanding more from support personnel, including secretaries, according to the International Association of Administrative Professionals. Because they are asking more of secretaries, organizations are also increasing salaries.

FOR MORE INFO

For information on certification and on seminars and workshops, contact:
International Association of Administrative Professionals
10502 NW Ambassador Drive
PO Box 20404
Kansas City, MO 64195-0404
Tel: 816-891-6600
Web: http://www.iaap-hq.org

For information on training, contact:
Arlington Career Institute
901 Avenue K
Grand Prairie, Texas 75050
Tel: 800-394-5445
Email: ACRI1@swbell.net
Web: http://www.themetro.com/aci

RELATED JOBS

Legal Secretaries
Medical Assistants
Medical Record Technicians
Secretaries

Medical Technologists

Med Tech Specialties

Some medical laboratory technologists specialize. Those who work in the **hematology** department analyze cells from blood and bone marrow. They diagnose and monitor patients with anemia, leukemia, and other blood infections. In **serology,** technologists do tests for syphillis, rheumatoid arthritis, and lupus. Technologists in **microbiology** identify bacteria, viruses, and fungi that cause disease. In **urinalysis,** technologists test patients' urine to identify infections, kidney or liver disease, and pregnancy by analyzing the presence of certain chemicals.

What Medical Technologists Do

Medical technologists do laboratory tests to help physicians find, diagnose, and treat diseases. They are usually supervised by a *pathologist,* a medical doctor who specializes in finding the causes and characteristics of diseases.

Technologists stain and mount slides with samples and examine them under a microscope. This allows them to see disease or damage to the cells. Medical technologists perform blood counts and skin tests. They do blood tests, including tests to determine blood types. They maintain blood supplies to be used for transfusions. Technologists also use microscopes to examine body fluids and tissue samples for bacteria, viruses, or other organisms. They test samples of blood and urine to find out if drugs, chemicals, or poisons are present.

Technologists prepare samples of tissue

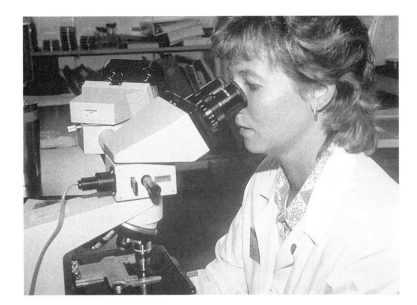

A medical technologist examines a blood sample for the presence of bacteria.

and bone for pathologists to examine. The samples are preserved in a variety of ways, including freezing. Many times an abnormal growth is sent to a laboratory while a patient is in surgery. The technologist tests the growth to see if it is cancerous. The test results help the surgeon decide how to proceed with the operation. Technologists also help pathologists determine the cause of death and preserve organs for later examination. Some medical technologists do research on new drugs. Others help to improve methods of laboratory testing.

Medical technologists must pay close attention to detail. They must be good at observing and analyzing. They must stay calm under pressure. Most medical tech-

EXPLORING

• **Learn how to use a microscope. Learn how to prepare samples on slides for viewing under a microscope.**

• **Work on science projects and experiments that involve lab work and chemistry. Get familiar with lab equipment and procedures. Ask for help from your science teacher.**

WORDS TO LEARN

Blood bank: The lab area where technicians draw blood from donors. Technicians also separate, identify, and match its components.

Cytology: The study of cells.

Hematology: The lab area that counts, describes, and identifies cells in blood and other body fluids.

Histology: The study of the structure and function of normal and abnormal tissue.

Immunology: The branch of medicine dealing with the body's ability to cope with infections.

Pathology: The study of the nature of disease, its structure, and the changes produced by disease.

Virology: the study of viruses and viral diseases.

nologists work in hospitals. Others work in laboratories, clinics, public health agencies, physicians' offices, drug companies, and research institutions.

Education and Training

High school courses in mathematics, biology, chemistry, physics, and computer science are important for a career in medical technology. You must earn a bachelor's degree for most jobs. To earn this degree, you must complete three years of college studies and a 12-month program in a school of medical technology. These schools usually are associated with colleges and universities. Some technologists earn master's degrees or doctorates in this field. They may get jobs in teaching and research.

Technologists may be certified by various organizations. To receive certification, you must pass examinations. Certain states require technologists to be licensed.

Earnings

Medical technologists earn average starting salaries of about $25,000 a year. Experienced technologists average $30,700 a year. Beginning medical technologists who work for the federal government receive annual salaries of about $23,000, depending on school records, education, and experience. The average for all medical technologists in the federal government is $32,000.

Outlook

Employment in this field is expected to grow as fast as the average through 2006. Because of a general shortage in hospital staffs, there will be a number of openings for medical technologists. The greatest demand will most likely be in independent medical laboratories. There also will be job opportunities in physicians' offices, clinics, in teaching, and in research.

FOR MORE INFO

For career information, contact the following organizations:

American Medical Technologists
710 Higgins Road
Park Ridge, IL 60068
Tel: 847-823-5169
Web: http://www.amt1.com

American Society for Clinical Laboratory Science
7910 Woodmont, Suite 530
Bethesda, MD 20814
Tel: 301-657-2768
Web: http://www.ascls.org

Acccrediting Bureau of Health Education Schools
3132 US 20 West
Elkhart, IN 46514
Tel: 219-295-0214

RELATED JOBS

Biologists
Biomedical Equipment Technicians
Pharmacologists
Pathologists
Physicians

Nurse Assistants

Where They Work

Over one-half of nurse assistants are employed in nursing homes. Others work in:

Hospitals

Halfway houses

Retirement centers

Homes for people with disabilities

Private homes

What Nurse Assistants Do

Nurse assistants, also called *nurse aides, orderlies,* or *hospital attendants,* take care of the personal needs of patients. They work in hospitals, nursing homes, mental health facilities, and drug and alcohol rehabilitation centers. Their duties vary according to the place they work and the kind of patients they care for. In general, they help move patients, assist in patients' exercise and nutrition needs, and oversee patients' personal hygiene. They are supervised by registered nurses.

Nurse assistants answer patients' message bells. They serve and feed patients' meals. They make beds, help patients to dress, undress, and bathe, give massages, take temperatures, bring and empty bedpans, help patients get out of bed and walk, and take them places in wheelchairs or on stretchers. Some aspects of the job are difficult and unpleasant, such as assisting a resident

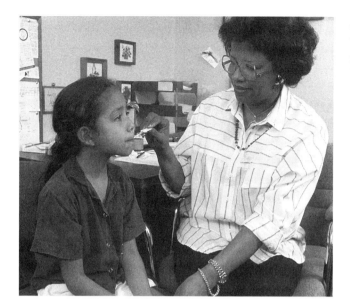

A nurse assistant takes a young patient's temperature.

with elimination and cleaning up after a patient who has vomited. Nurse assistants in nursing homes and long-term health care facilities usually have much more contact with the patients than other members of the staff, and they often develop positive ongoing relationships with the people under their care.

Nurse assistants must sometimes work with disturbed, confused, anxious, or even violent patients. These experiences can be emotionally exhausting for the assistants, who must at always act professionally and maintain a calm, patient, and sympathetic manner.

Today there are about 1.4 million nurse assistants in the United States and about

EXPLORING

• Offer to care for a sick grandparent or neighbor. You can help an adult run errands, do laundry, or prepare meals.

• Learn about first aid, nutrition, exercise, and massage.

half of them work in nursing homes.

Education and Training

Most employers prefer to hire people with a high school diploma. Some high schools work with local hospitals or nursing homes to offer health care courses.

Most nursing homes and hospitals offer on-the-job training, which can last anywhere from two weeks to three months. There are training courses available at community colleges and vocational schools that teach basic nursing skills and prepare you for the state certification exam. You must be certified to work in a nursing home. In some states you must be certi-

NURSE ASSISTANT SHORTAGE

Marsha Austin reports in *The Denver Business Journal* that there is a serious shortage of nurse assistants in the Denver area. They are being drawn to jobs in casinos and retail stores where the pay is about the same, but the work is less physically and emotionally demanding.

Hospitals are offering higher pay to attract nurse assistants, but many nursing homes can't afford to pay much more than minimum wage. Enrollment in Certified Nursing Assistant programs is way down. "This critical shortage of nurses' aides threatens to leave Denver's elderly, disabled, and chronically ill without basic health care and the tight labor market is to blame," says Austin.

fied no matter where you work.

Earnings

Salaries for nurse assistants are not high, but all assistants earn at least minimum wage. Wages for nurse assistants range from $14,500 to $18,000 a year. Nursing homes pay certified nurse assistants salaries of about $13,000 a year. Wages in hospitals are slightly higher depending upon your level of experience. Since health care facilities operate around the clock, assistants work shifts on evenings, nights, holidays, and weekends. They often earn overtime pay.

Outlook

Job prospects for nurse assistants look excellent through 2006. Though fewer aides will be hired by hospitals, many more will be needed by long-term health care facilities and nursing homes. As our population ages, geriatric nurse assistants will be needed to care for elderly patients.

FOR MORE INFO

For information about careers as nursing assistants, contact:
American Health Care Association
1201 L Street, NW
Washington, DC 20005

American Hospital Association
Division of Nursing
1 East Franklin Street, Suite 27
Chicago, IL 60606
Tel: 312-422-3000

Career Nurse Assistant Program, Inc.
3577 Easton Road
Norton, OH 44203
Tel: 330-825-9342
Web: http://www.cna~network.org

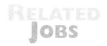

RELATED JOBS

Advanced Practice Nurses
Home Health Care Aides
Hospice Workers
Medical Assistants
Nurses

Nurses

Florence Nightingale (1820-1910) was a strong influence on the development of nursing as a profession. She dedicated her life to improving conditions in hospitals, beginning in an army hospital during the Crimean War. In the United States, many of Nightingale's ideas were practiced during the Civil War. The care, however, was provided by concerned people rather than by trained nurses.

The first school of nursing in the United States was started in Boston in 1873. In 1938, New York State passed the first state law to require that practical nurses be licensed.

Education standards for nurses have been improving constantly ever since. Today's nurse is a highly educated, licensed health care professional. Training programs are offered throughout the country, and all states have laws concerning training standards and licensing.

What Nurses Do

Nurses care for people who are sick, injured, or mentally ill. Nurses have a wide variety of duties. They comfort and assist patients, give treatments and medication, record patients' progress, and prepare equipment. Depending on their training, nurses also assist physicians and surgeons in medical procedures and supervise or teach other nursing staff. Nurses can specialize in many different areas.

General duty nurses work as part of a health care team. The team determines a patient's condition and decides on a health care plan. Nurses take patients' blood pressure, temperature, and pulse. They give medications. They note the patient's condition and symptoms. They change dressings, get patients ready for surgery, and complete any other duties that require skill and an understanding of the patient's needs.

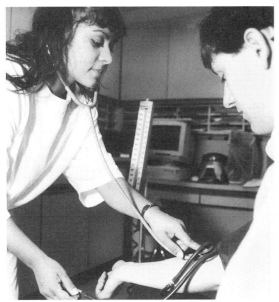

A nurse takes a patient's blood pressure.

Surgical nurses assist surgeons during operations. *Maternity nurses* help in the delivery room and take care of newborns in the nursery. They teach mothers how to feed and care for their babies. *Private duty nurses* work in hospitals and in patients' homes. They are employed by the patient or the patient's family, and they work under the supervision of the patient's physician. *Occupational health nurses* work in plants or factories. They give first aid treatment in emergencies. They also offer preventive and educational nursing services. *School nurses* supervise the student clinic, treat minor ailments and injuries, and give general health advice. *Hospice nurses* work with the terminally ill. They may treat patients in hospitals or hospice facilities, but often

EXPLORING

• **Read books about famous nurses, such as Clara Barton, Elizabeth Fry, Edith Cavell, and Florence Nightingale.**

• **Talk to your school nurse or local public health nurse about their jobs.**

• **Visit your local hospital to see what the work environment is like.**

• **Volunteer to work at a hospital, community health center, or even the local Red Cross chapter.**

travel to patients' homes to offer treatment.

Licensed practical nurses (L.P.N.s), sometimes called *licensed vocational nurses,* perform the basic duties of nursing, including general patient care, the giving of medication, and clerical duties. They work under the supervision of *registered nurses* (R.N.s) and physicians. *Advanced practice nurses* are nurses who have received training beyond the R.N. level.

Education and Training

High school classes in biology, chemistry, health, mathematics, and social science provide a good background for nursing.

L.P.N.s usually complete a one-year educational program after high school. All states require you to pass an examination to be licensed. You must graduate from an approved school of practical nursing before you take this examination.

To become an R.N., you must choose one of three training programs. An associate's degree program is a two-year program offered at a community or junior college. A diploma program is a three-year program offered at hospitals and nursing schools. Bachelor's degree programs are four- or five-year programs offered at colleges and universities. You must earn a bachelor's degree in nursing for most supervisory and administrative positions, for jobs in public health agencies, and for admission to graduate nursing programs. A master's degree is usually necessary to prepare for a nursing specialty or to teach. For some specialties, such as nursing research, you must earn a Ph.D.

Earnings

Registered nurses earn about $36,244 a year. R.N.s who work

in nursing homes earn about $32,968 a year. The average annual salary for nurses in federal government agencies is about $26,100. L.P.N.s earn about $24,336 a year.

Outlook

In 1996, there were nearly 2 million nurses employed in the United States, making nursing the largest of all health care occupations. Employment in nursing homes is expected to grow much faster than the average in the next ten years. The U.S. Department of Labor says that registered nurses will be one of the top 25 occupations with fastest growth, high pay, and low unemployment. The department says there will be about 425,000 additional jobs available by 2006.

Nurses wil be needed to staff the growing number of nursing homes. Many nurses also will be needed to staff outpatient facilities, such as Health Maintenance Organizations, group medical practices, and

FOR MORE INFO

For information on nursing careers, contact the following organizations.

American Nurses' Association
600 Maryland Avenue, SW, Suite 100W
Washington, DC 20024-2571
Tel: 800-274-4ANA
Web: http://www.nursingworld.org

American Association of Colleges of Nursing
One Dupont Circle, Suite 530
Washington, DC 20036
Tel: 202-463-6930
Web: http://www.aacn.nche.edu

National Association for Practical Nurse Education and Service, Inc.
1400 Spring Street, Suite 310
Silver Spring, MD 20910
Tel: 301-588-2491
Email: napnes@aol.com
Web: http://www.aoa.dhhs.gov/aoa

outpatient surgery centers.

Two-thirds of all nursing positions are found in hospitals. But because of cost cutting, increased nurse's work load, and fast growth of outpatient services, hospital nursing jobs will experience slower than average growth.

Nutritionists

What Nutritionists Do

Nutritionists are experts on food, diet, and nutrition. They provide people with foods that will improve or maintain their health, and they teach people about nutrition. They usually work in hospitals, schools, restaurants, and hotels—any place where food is served or where people have special nutritional needs. Some nutritionists are dietitians. *Dietitians* have completed the strict training and testing requirements of the American Dietetic Association (ADA). Nutritionists usually specialize in one particular area.

Clinical nutritionists plan and supervise the preparation of diets for specific patients. They work for hospitals and retirement homes. In many cases, their patients cannot eat certain foods for medical reasons, such as diabetes or liver failure. Nutritionists must see that these patients receive nourishing meals. Clinical nutritionists work closely with doctors, who advise them regarding their

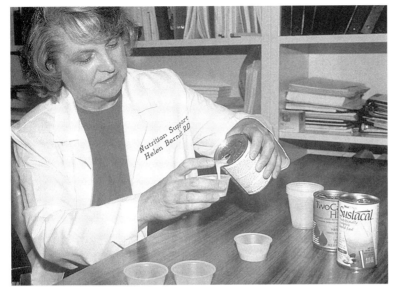

A dietitian prepares to test a variety of nutritional supplements to see if they meet her exacting standards.

patients' health and the foods that the patients cannot eat. Clinical nutritionists often teach the public about nutritional principles.

Although most nutritionists do some kind of teaching in their work, *teaching nutritionists* specialize in education. They usually work for hospitals, and they may teach full-time or part-time. Sometimes, teaching nutritionists also perform other tasks, such as running a food-service operation, especially in small colleges. In some cases, teaching nutritionists also do research.

Consultant nutritionists work with schools, restaurants, grocery-store chains, manufacturers of food-service

EXPLORING

• **Read books about healthy diet and nutrition. Many cookbooks that feature healthy recipes have sections on nutrition.**

• **Start collecting healthy recipes.**

• **Prepare a healthy meal for your family once a week.**

WHAT DO DIETETIC TECHNICIANS DO?

Dietetic technicians work in two areas: food-service management and nutrition care of individuals, also known as clinical nutrition. They usually work on a team, under the direction of a dietitian. Most technicians work for hospitals and nursing homes. Some, however, work for health agencies such as public health departments or neighborhood health centers.

Technicians in food-service management work in kitchens, overseeing the actual food preparation. Some supervise dietetic aides who serve food to patients in the cafeteria and in their hospital rooms. Technicians sometimes develop recipes as well as diet plans for patients. They also may help patients select their menus. Some keep track of food items on hand, order supplies, and supervise food storage.

Technicians in clinical nutrition work under the supervision of a dietitian. They interview patients about their eating habits and the foods they like. They give this information to the dietitian, along with reports on each patient's progress. Technicians teach patients and their families about good nutrition.

Education and Training: Dietetic technicians must have a high school diploma and complete a two-year program approved by the American Dietetic Association that leads to an associate's degree.

Earnings: Beginning technicians earn between $15,000 and $20,000 a year. Workers with 10 to 15 years of experience may earn between $20,000 and $25,000 a year. Those at the top of the pay scale earn between $30,000 and $35,000.

Outlook: The outlook for dietetic technicians, especially those who are certified, is generally very good through 2006.

equipment, drug companies, and private companies of various kinds. Some consultants work with athletes and sports teams. They help improve athletes' performance and extend the length of their careers.

Research nutritionists work for government organizations, universities, hospitals, drug companies, and manufacturers. They try to improve existing food products or find alternatives to unhealthy foods.

Education and Training

Most nutritionists have at least two years of college-level training in nutrition, food service, or another related subject. To become a Registered Dietitian (R.D.), you must have a bachelor's degree. Then you must complete a practice program that takes six to 12 months, and pass an exam.

For many positions in institutions, you must be an R.D. If you want to teach, do research, or work in public health, you will need one or more advanced degrees.

FOR MORE INFO

The ADA is the single best source of information about careers in dietetics. Its Web site is an excellent resource that provides detailed information and links to other organizations and resources.

American Dietetic Association
216 West Jackson Boulevard, Suite 800
Chicago, IL 60606
Tel: 800-877-1600, ext. 4897
Email: network@eatright.org
Web: http://www.eatright.org

The ASNS is a good source of educational and career information.
American Society for Nutritional Sciences
9650 Rockville Pike
Bethesda, MD 20814
Tel: 301-530-7050
Web: http://www.faseb.org/asns

Earnings

The ADA says that most entry-level R.D.s make between $25,000 and $45,000 a year. Many experienced R.D.s make more than $50,000 yearly, and some of them make $70,000 or more.

Outlook

According to the U.S. Department of Labor's 1998-1999 *Occupational Outlook Handbook,* employment of dietitians and nutritionists will have average growth through 2006. As the population ages, more positions for nutritionists will become available.

Orthotists and Prosthetists

In the Beginning

Throughout history people have tried to replace lost limbs and support weak body parts. Braces, splints, and other corrective devices have been used since prehistoric times. Devices used during the Middle Ages included splints made out of leather for hips and legs, special shoes, and solid metal hands.

Some of the most dramatic advances made in the fields of prosthetics and orthotics have occurred during and after major wars. After World War II, for example, prosthetists discovered new lightweight plastics that could be used to make artificial arms and hands. There is a great need for skilled workers in this field. More than 125,000 people lose a limb each year to illness or injury. Thousands of others have some sort of physical disability that requires orthotic assistance.

What Orthotists and Prosthetists Do

Prosthetists make artificial limbs for patients who have lost limbs. *Orthotists* make braces to support weak limbs or help correct a physical problem, such as a deformed spine.

Physicians refer patients to an orthotist or a prosthetist. Orthotists and prosthetists first examine their patients to determine what type of device is needed. A prosthetist uses tapes and rulers to measure limbs or stumps carefully. Orthotists also take detailed measurements for braces.

The device must fit the patient well so that it will work properly without causing irritation. Orthotists and prosthetists always try to design the most comfortable, useful, and natural-looking device possible. Each device is specially designed to match an individual's body. A process called *cineplasty* is sometimes used. In this process, a control is

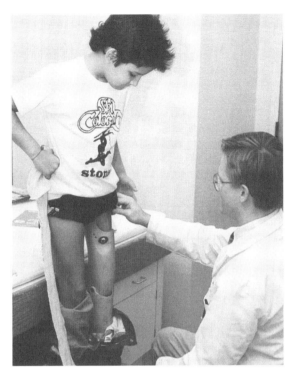

attached to the patient's actual muscle. This allows the patient to better control movement.

Orthotists and prosthetists work with physicians and therapists to design and make these special devices. These devices require all sorts of materials such as wood, foam, fabric, leather, metal, and plastic. Orthotists and prosthetists use both hand tools and power tools to shape the parts and assemble them.

Once the devices are made, prosthetists and orthotists fit them to their patients. They need to be creative in designing these devices and sympathetic in work-

EXPLORING

• Teachers and counselors may be able to arrange for you to visit a hospital, clinic, or rehabilitation center so you can talk with people in this field.

• Read all you can about science, especially physics, and engineering.

• Try to invent machines or tools of all kinds.

• Read about robotics.

WORDS TO LEARN

AFO: An abbreviation for "ankle-foot orthosis," which is a brace supporting this area.

KAFO: An abbreviation for "knee-ankle-foot orthosis," which is a brace supporting this area.

Myoelectrics: The technology using electrical impulses from muscles to trigger a motorized part in a prosthesis, which then causes the prosthesis to move.

Orthosis: A device applied to the outside of the body to immobilize or assist the motion of a specific part. An orthosis is usually called a brace.

Plaster cast model: A form of a patient's body part, poured in plaster from the impressions taken by an orthotist or prosthetist.

Prosthesis: A device used in place of a limb that is partially or completely missing

Reliefs and build-ups: Pads of specified thickness that are placed in certain parts of the orthotic device.

Thermoforming: Using heat and sometimes pressure to shape a substance such as plastic.

ing with their patients. They must make any alterations the patients need to comfortably wear the devices. After fitting, they will also help patients learn to use the artificial limbs or braces.

Prosthetists and orthotists usually work for hospitals and rehabilitation centers. Some set up private practice.

Education and Training

High school courses in the sciences, psychology, mechanical drawing, and shop will help you prepare for work in prosthetics or orthotics. To become a prosthetist or an orthotist, you must go to college and earn a bachelor's degree. In college, you will study science and engineering. You will also practice making and fitting devices in laboratories.

A prosthetist or orthotist who has graduated from college

and worked in the field for one or two years can try to earn certification from the American Board for Certification in Orthotics and Prosthetics. To earn certification, you must pass the board's exam. Although certification is not required, those who are certified usually have better job opportunities and make more money.

Earnings

Starting salaries are about $27,500 a year for certified orthotists and prosthetists. Those with more experience earn around $54,000 a year. Those who are certified, have a great deal of experience, and work in large hospitals can earn more than $60,000 a year. Those who are not certified make less money.

Outlook

The orthotics and prosthetics field should grow in the next 10 years. This will be due to new developments in the field, the increasing number of older peo-

FOR MORE INFO

For information on careers and educational opportunities in orthotics and prosthetics, contact:
Orthotists and Prosthetists Headquarters
1650 King Street, Suite 500
Alexandria, VA 22314
Tel: 703-836-7114

For information on orthotic and prosthetic careers with the U.S. government, contact:
Veterans Health Administration
810 Vermont Avenue, NW
Washington, DC 20420
Tel: 202-273-5782

For information on becoming a certified orthotist or prosthetist, contact:
American Board for Certification in Orthotics and Prosthetics
1650 King Street, Suite 500
Alexandria, VA 22314
Tel: 703-836-7114
Web: http://www.opoffice.org

ple, and changes in insurance coverage.

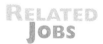

RELATED JOBS

Biomedical Engineers
Occupational Therapists
Physical Therapists

Physical Therapists

What Physical Therapists Do

Physical therapists help people who have been injured or ill to recover and relearn daily living skills, such as walking, eating and bathing. They work with elderly people who have had accidents or strokes. They also work with children who have birth defects or disabilities and athletes who have been injured.

It can be very rewarding for a physical therapist when a person is able to perform an activity they once routinely did. Physical therapy helps burn victims avoid abnormal scarring and loss of movement. It helps patients with heart problems improve endurance. And it can help cancer patients relieve their pain.

Physical therapists first evaluate new patients to decide what treatment would help them. The therapist works as part of a health care team that may include the patient's physician or surgeon, nurse,

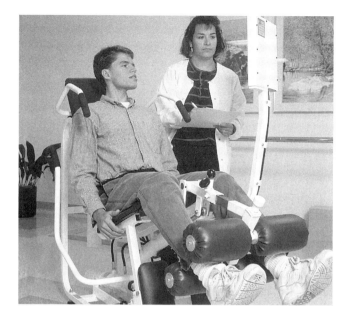

A physical therapist monitors the physical conditioning and progress of her patient.

occupational therapist, and psychologist. After setting treatment goals for the patient, the physical therapist decides which methods to use.

If a patient has muscle damage in a leg, for example, the physical therapist may move the muscle through different motions and watch how the patient stands and walks to decide whether the patient needs braces or specific exercises. Other treatments often prescribed by therapists include hydrotherapy (the use of water in treatment), paraffin baths, infrared lamps, heating pads, ice, ultrasound or electrical current.

Depending on the patient's injury or disability, therapy may take place over a few

EXPLORING

• **Ask your teacher to arrange a visit to a physical therapy department at a hospital to see physical therapists at work.**

• **Read books on these subjects:**

  Massage

  Occupational therapy

  Arts therapy

  Anatomy

weeks, months, or even years. Physical therapists also teach patients and their families so that they can continue care at home.

Many physical therapists work in hospitals. Others work in private physical therapy offices, nursing homes, rehabilitation centers, schools, homes, sports medicine clinics, and industrial clinics.

Education and Training

To prepare for a physical therapy career, you should take high school courses in health, biology, chemistry, and physics.

WHAT DO PHYSICAL THERAPY ASSISTANTS DO?

Physical therapy assistants help physical therapists in a variety of techniques, such as exercise, massage, heat, and water therapy. These treatments help restore physical function in people with injury, birth defects, or disease.

Physical therapy assistants work directly under the supervision of physical therapists. They help patients improve activities required in their daily lives, such as walking, climbing, and moving from one place to another. The assistants observe patients during treatments, record the patients' responses and progress, and report these to the physical therapist. They fit patients for and teach them to use braces, artificial limbs, crutches, canes, walkers, wheelchairs, and other devices. They may make physical measurements to record patients' range of motion, length and girth of body parts, and vital signs.

Education and Training: Physical therapy assistants must graduate from an accredited, two-year physical therapy assistant program. These programs are offered at junior and community colleges.

Earnings: Beginning assistants earn between $20,000 and $24,000 a year. Experienced assistants earn between $25,000 and $30,000 a year.

Outlook: Employment prospects are good through 2006. Job growth is expected to be 80 percent.

Physical therapists must earn at least a bachelor's degree. Many earn postgraduate degrees. After graduation from a program, therapists must pass an exam to become licensed. After a few years of work experience, you can earn a specialist certification. The American Board of Physical Therapy Specialties certifies physical therapists who show advanced knowledge in a specialty area. These specialties include cardiopulmonary, geriatric, pediatric, and sports physical therapy.

Earnings

Physical therapists earn average salaries of $39,364 a year. According to the American Therapy Association, hospital therapists earn an average of $48,000 a year. The average for therapists working for the federal government is $26,400 a year.

Outlook

Physical therapy is one of the fastest-growing professions in the United States. In 1996, 115,000 physical therapists

FOR MORE INFO

The American Physical Therapy Association offers a brochure entitled "A Future in Physical Therapy" as well as other general career information.
American Physical Therapy Association
1111 North Fairfax Street
Alexandria, VA 22314
Tel: 800-999-2782
Web: http://www.apta.org

were employed. About 25 percent worked part-time. The Bureau of Labor Statistics predicts growth of about 75 percent through 2006.

As the number of middle-aged and elderly Americans grows, more people develop medical conditions that require physical therapy. As people live longer and more trauma victims and newborns with defects survive, the need for physical therapists rises.

Physicians

The first great physician was Hippocrates, a Greek who lived almost 2,500 years ago. He developed theories about medicine and the anatomy of the human body. But Hippocrates is remembered today for a set of medical ethics that still influences medical practice. The Hippocratic oath that he administered to his disciples is still given in a slightly different variation to new physicians today. His 87 essays on medicine, known as the "Hippocratic Collection," are believed to be the first record of early medical theory and practice. Hippocratic physicians believed that health was maintained by a proper balance of four "humors" in the body: blood, phlegm, black bile, and yellow bile.

What Physicians Do

Physicians examine patients' bodies, determine if they are sick or well, and decide on any treatment they need. Physicians must know all about how the body works and, when it does not work properly, they must know the possible ways to repair it.

Most physicians work in private practice. They see patients by appointment in their offices and in hospitals if they have serious illnesses. Many physicians are *general* or *family practitioners* who provide medical services to families and individuals of all ages and both sexes, usually on a regular basis. They perform routine check-ups, treat patients when they are sick or injured, and give advice about diet, exercise, and other health-related matters. Family practitioners can diagnose and treat most ailments. Some family practitioners set broken bones, deliver babies, or perform minor surgery.

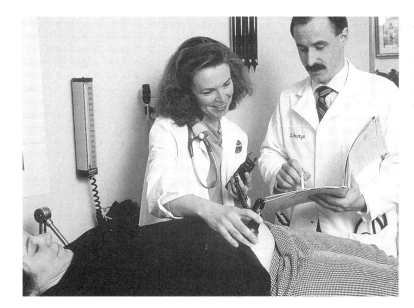

A physician gives instuctions to his assistant as she performs a routine examination on a pregnant woman.

When the patient's problem is severe or unusual, the family practitioner sends the patient to a physician who specializes in that disorder. For example, *cardiologists* take care of patients with heart disease. *Dermatologists* treat diseases and problems of the skin, hair, and nails. *Internists* treat diseases and injuries of the internal organs, including the lungs, stomach and kidneys. *Pediatricians* care for children from birth to approximately the teenage years. *Gynecologists* and *obstetricians* are concerned with the health of a woman's reproductive system. They treat diseases and also provide care before, during, and after childbirth. *Surgeons* perform operations that repair injuries, help prevent disease, and improve the health of a patient.

EXPLORING

• In high school, you might be able to volunteer at a local hospital, clinic, or nursing home. This is a good way to learn what it's like to work around other health care professionals and patients.

• Read as much as possible about the profession, including books on anatomy, medicines, diseases, health and fitness, and nutrition.

• Take a class in first aid and CPR.

Education and Training

You must study and train for many years before you can practice medicine. If you want to become a doctor, you should take high school college-preparatory courses, including English, a foreign language, social studies, mathematics, biology, chemistry, physics, and computer science. Also while in high school, volunteering in a hospital or medical office is good experience. After high school, you must attend college. A pre-med program is ideal, but you can major in any subject. It is important, though, to take science courses.

After college, you must go to medical school. In the first two years of medical school, you will learn about human anatomy, physiology, human cells, and prescription drugs. During the last two years, you will spend your time in a hospital and become part of a medical team. Beginning with basic tasks, you learn medical skills by practicing them under the close supervision of licensed physicians. You may take personal histories from patients, make diagnoses, and perform

Is THERE A DOCTOR IN THE HOUSE?

Before the 1960s, doctors often visited patients in their homes. They carried a black bag full of tools and medicines. Since then, the tools of the trade have become too high-tech to fit into a black bag, so patients have had to go to physicians' offices. Now high-tech equipment is getting smaller and doctors are able to fit just about everything they need into a car. And they are reviving the old practice of house calls.

According to the American Medical Association, house calls may be the best medicine for patients. Home visits are cheaper than the emergency room. Another benefit is that the doctor can tell much more about the patient's life and perhaps see the effect of environmental or emotional factors on the patient's health.

laboratory tests. You also learn about medical specialties, such as pediatrics, psychiatry, obstetrics and gynecology, surgery, and family practice.

Once you receive your medical degree (M.D.), you must pass a test to be licensed to practice. Most physicians then complete from one to three more years of training, usually as hospital residents or interns. If you wish to become a specialist, you will spend another three to five years in training.

Earnings

Physicians have among the highest earnings of any occupation. According to the American Medical Association, the median income for all physicians is about $160,000 a year. The median income of radiologists is $230,000. General surgeons earn about $225,000. Family practitioners earn $124,000. Anesthesiologists earn $230,000, and emergency medicine physicians earn about $170,000.

FOR MORE INFO

For career information, contact:
American Academy of Family Physicians
8880 Ward Parkway
Kansas City, MO 64114
Tel: 816-333-9700
Web: http://www.aafp.org

American Medical Association
515 North State Street
Chicago, IL 60610
Tel: 312-464-5000
Web: http://www.ama-assn.org

For a list of accredited U.S. and Canadian medical schools and other education information, contact:
Association of American Medical Colleges
2450 N Street, NW
Washington, DC 20037
Tel: 202-828-0400
Web: http://www.aamc.org

Outlook

The outlook for physicians is excellent. The occupation is expected to grow faster than the average through 2006. Population growth, especially among the elderly, will increase the demand for physicians.

Psychiatrists

Phobias are extreme or abnormal fears. Approximately 4 to 5 percent of Americans have one or more significant phobias in a given year. Here are just a few:

Achluophobia
Fear of darkness

Acrophobia
Fear of heights

Agoraphobia
Fear of open spaces

Ceraunophobia
Fear of thunder

Claustrophobia
Fear of enclosed or narrow spaces

Cynophobia
Fear of dogs

Glossophobia
Fear of speaking in public

Hydrophobia
Fear of water

Polyphobia
Fear of many things

Scolionophobia
Fear of school

What Psychiatrists Do

Psychiatrists are physicians who treat and prevent mental illness. They work with clients who might have feelings of anger or fear, or people who are so confused that they have completely lost touch with reality. Psychiatrists use a variety of methods to treat patients. They might discuss problems, prescribe medicine, or combine discussions, medication, and other types of therapy.

Mental illness has several possible causes. A mental problem might be caused by a physical disorder. It might be caused by a person's inability to handle stress and conflict. Some disorders are only temporary while others last a long time. People with mental problems cannot do certain things because of the way they think, feel, or act. Whenever possible, psychiatrists help these people overcome their problems and lead happier lives.

To determine the cause of a mental illness, psychiatrists interview patients and give them complete physical examinations. To understand patients, a psychiatrist must learn about important events in their lives and any strong feelings or opinions they have towards others. Many times a psychiatrist can improve a patient's condition by helping him or her understand why a problem has occurred. Together, the psychiatrist and patient then find other ways for the patient to think and behave. This process is called *psychotherapy*. In cases where discussing a problem is not enough, or when serious mental problems are caused by a brain disorder, a psychiatrist may prescribe medication.

Education and Training

The psychiatrist's work can be emotionally demanding. Psychiatrists spend much of their time with people who are depressed and angry. Some patients may even be suicidal.

You need many years of schooling and experience to become a psychiatrist. After you graduate from a four-year college, you must enter a four-year program at a medical school. These programs provide extensive training in anatomy, biolo-

EXPLORING

• **Read all you can about psychiatry.** *Career Planning for Psychiatrists* (1995), edited by Kathleen M. Mogul, M.D. and Leah J. Dickstein, M.D., is a comprehensive guide to the various career opportunities available in psychiatry.

• **Talk with your school counselors and ask them for information about psychiatry careers.**

FAMOUS PSYCHIATRISTS

The greatest advances in psychiatric treatment came in the latter part of the 19th century. **Emil Kraepelin** (1856-1926), a German psychiatrist, made an important contribution when he developed a classification system for mental illnesses that is still used for diagnosis today. **Sigmund Freud** (1856-1939), the famous Viennese psychiatrist, developed techniques for analyzing human behavior that have strongly influenced the practice of modern psychiatry. Freud first lectured in the United States in 1909. Swiss psychiatrist **Carl Jung** (1875-1961), a former associate of Freud's, revolutionized the field with his theory of a collective unconscious.

you can begin to practice as a psychiatrist, you must pass oral and written exams given by the American Board of Psychiatry and Neurology.

Earnings

Psychiatrists' earnings depend on the kind of practice they have and its location, their experience, and the number of patients they treat. Like other physicians, their average income is among the highest of any occupation.

gy, medical practices, and other subjects. After graduating from medical school, you must pass exams to become a medical doctor. You then complete at least four additional years of training in the treatment of the mentally ill. You study medical practices, but mostly you train on-the-job at a psychiatric hospital. You are closely supervised by experienced psychiatrists during this time. Before

Average income for psychiatrists is $137,200 a year, according to the American Medical Association. Psychiatrists in private practice earn about $148,800 a year. Salaried employees working for hospitals or other health care institutions earn an average of $127,500 a year.

Outlook

During the next decade there

will be a strong demand for skilled psychiatrists. Growing population and increasing life span mean more people will need psychiatric care. Rising incomes allow more people to afford treatment. Higher educational levels make more people aware of the importance of mental health care. A shortage of psychiatrists, especially for children and in rural areas, will keep job opportunities bright through the year 2006.

FOR MORE INFO

For information on psychiatry, contact:
American Medical Association
515 North State Street
Chicago, IL 60610
Tel: 312-464-5000
Web: http://www.ama-assn.org

American Psychiatric Association
1400 K Street, NW
Washington, DC 20005
Tel: 202-682-6000

National Mental Health Association
1021 Prince Street
Alexandria, VA 22314-2971
Tel: 703-684-5968
Web: http://www.com/pfalzgraf/nmha.html

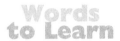
Words to Learn

Neurosis: An emotional disorder that arises due to unresolved conflicts. Anxiety is often the main characteristic.
Phobia: A persistent, unrealistic fear of an object or situation.
Psychoanalysis: A method of treating mental disorders by bringing unconscious fears and conflicts into the conscious mind.
Psychosis: A major mental disorder, in which the personality is seriously disorganized and the person loses contact with reality.
Psychosomatic: A physical illness caused or made worse by a mental condition.
Psychotherapy: The treatment of mental disorders by psychological, rather than physical, means.

RELATED JOBS

Nurses
Physicians
Psychiatric Technicians
Psychologists

Glossary

accredited: Approved as meeting established standards for providing good training and education. This approval is usually given by an independent organization of professionals to a school or a program in a school. Compare **certified** and **licensed**.

apprentice: A person who is learning a trade by working under the supervision of a skilled worker. Apprentices often receive classroom instruction in addition to their supervised practical experience.

apprenticeship: 1. A program for training apprentices (see apprentice). 2. The period of time when a person is an apprentice. In highly skilled trades, apprenticeships may last three or four years.

associate's degree: An academic rank or title granted by a community or junior college or similar institution to graduates of a two-year program of education beyond high school.

bachelor's degree: An academic rank or title given to a person who has completed a four-year program of study at a college or university. Also called an undergraduate degree or baccalaureate.

certified: Approved as meeting established requirements for skill, knowledge, and experience in a particular field. People are certified by the organization of professionals in their field. Compare **accredited** and **licensed**.

community college: A public two-year college, attended by students who do not live at the college. Graduates of a community college receive an associate degree and may transfer to a four-year college or university to complete a bachelor's degree. Compare **junior college** and **technical college**.

diploma: A certificate or document given by a school to show that a person has completed a course or has graduated from the school.

doctorate: An academic rank or title (the highest) granted by a graduate school to a person who has completed a two- to three-year program after having received a master's degree.

fringe benefit: A payment or benefit to an employee in addition to regular wages or salary. Examples of fringe benefits include a pension, a paid vacation, and health or life insurance.

graduate school: A school that people may attend after they have received their bachelor's degree. People who complete an educational program at a graduate school earn a master's degree or a doctorate.

intern: An advanced student (usually one with at least some college training) in a professional field who is employed in a job that is intended to provide supervised practical experience for the student.

internship: 1. The position or job of an intern (see intern). 2. The period of time when a person is an intern.

junior college: A two-year college that offers courses like those in the first half of a four-year college program. Graduates of a junior college usually receive an associate degree and may transfer to a four-year college or university to complete a bachelor's degree. Compare **community college.**

liberal arts: The subjects covered by college courses that develop broad general knowledge rather than specific occupational skills. The liberal arts are often considered to include philosophy, literature and the arts, history, language, and some courses in the social sciences and natural ciences.

licensed: Having formal permission from the proper authority to carry out an activity that would be illegal without that permission. For example, a person may be licensed to practice medicine or to drive a car. Compare **certified**.

major: (in college) The academic field in which a student specializes and receives a degree.

master's degree: An academic rank or title granted by a graduate school to a person who has completed a one- or two-year program after having received a bachelor's degree.

pension: An amount of money paid regularly by an employer to a former employee after he or she retires from working.

private: 1. Not owned or controlled by the government (such as private industry or a private employment agency). 2. Intended only for a particular person or group; not open to all (such as a private road or a private club).

public: 1.Provided or operated by the government (such as a public library). 2. Open and available to everyone (such as a public meeting).

regulatory: Having to do with the rules and laws for carrying out an activity. A regulatory agency, for example, is a government organization that sets up required procedures for how certain things should be done.

scholarship: A gift of money to a student to help the student pay for further education.

social studies: Courses of study (such as civics, geography, and history) that deal with how human societies work.

starting salary: Salary paid to a newly hired employee. The starting salary is usually a smaller amount than is paid to a more experienced worker.

technical college: A private or public college offering two- or four-year programs in technical subjects. Technical colleges offer courses in both general and technical subjects and award associate degrees and bachelor's degrees.

technician: A worker with specialized practical training in a mechanical or scientific subject who works under the supervision of scientists, engineers, or other professionals. Technicians typically receive two years of college-level education after high school.

technologist: A worker in a mechanical or scientific field with more training than a technician. Technologists typically must have between two and four years of college-level education after high school.

undergraduate: A student at a college or university who has not yet received a degree.

undergraduate degree: See **bachelor's degree**.

union: An organization whose members are workers in a particular industry or company. The union works to gain better wages, benefits, and working conditions for its members. Also called a labor union or trade union.

vocational school: A public or private school that offers training in one or more skills or trades. Compare **technical school**.

wage: Money that is paid in return for work done, especially money paid on the basis of the number of hours or days worked.

Index of Job Titles

Health on the Web

Benny Goodsport
http://www.bennygoodsport.com/

Health Care Career Information
http://hml.org/CHIS/career.html

Hospital Tour
http://funrsc.fairfield.edu/~jfleitas/hospital.html

Human Anatomy Online
www.innerbody.com/htm/body.html

The Human Body
http://pen.pa.k12.ri.us/Curric/Science/Human1.htm

Kids' Food Cyber Club
http://www.kidsfood.org/kf_cyber.html

Kids' Health and Fitness
http://www.ced.appstate.edu/whs/goals2000/projects/fitness.htm

KidsHealth.org
http://kidshealth.org/index2.html

Nutrition Explorations
http://www.nutritionexplorations.org/kids_zone.html

Yuckiest Site on the Internet
www.yucky.com/